15

Tips for
Quitting
Antidepressants

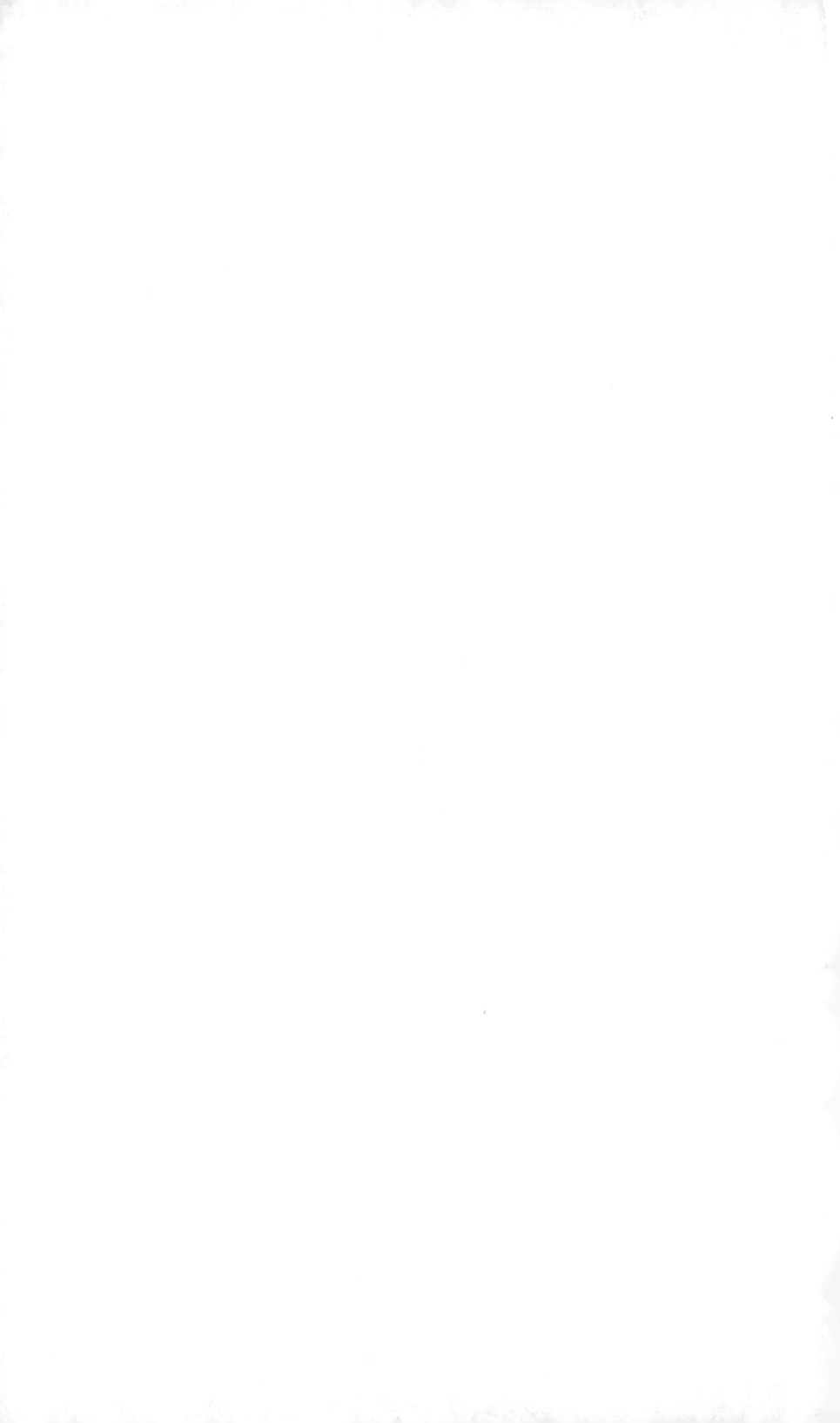

15

Tips for
Quitting
Antidepressants

WENDY MURRAY

ECCO QUA PRESS

Beverly, Massachusetts

15 Tips for Quitting Antidepressants

Copyright© 2016 Wendy Murray. All rights reserved. Printed in the United States of America. For information address Ecco Qua Press, Beverly, Massachusetts 01915.

Murray, Wendy.
15 Tips for Quitting Antidepressants / Wendy Murray.— 1st. ed.

ISBN: 978-1-4675-0069-2

Contents

Disclaimer

This book is not intended to replace medical advice. The information provided is simply an account of my personal journey to discontinue antidepressants highlighting key factors that worked for me. Please consult a healthcare professional before deciding the best course for your tapering.

Introduction

During the long days – weeks – months – and, yes, years of my own efforts to get off antidepressants I scoured internet forums looking for success stories, and there weren't many. More than the need to know who, if anyone, succeeded at this, I was desperate for encouragement and guidance as to how I myself might succeed. During the two years it took to finally navigate the journey off these meds (with three different attempts), help came to me only in bits and snatches that I gleaned from random postings on a variety of forums I found online.

It is my hope that this short book can serve as your encouragement and your guide as I recount the multi-faceted strategies I employed that finally paid off in success, at long last, in getting off and being free of antidepressant medication.

My story is not going to be your story in every excruciating detail. Every person's tapering journey is as unique as his or her brain chemistry. But it will bear similarities and there will be resonance. The hallmarks of this struggle are fairly similar (alas) among those who undertake it. In this regard, this book will ring true to you in your struggle and, I hope, will lend you aid.

Some of the material you find herein appears in some form on my website and blog, *Surviving SSRIs* (www.survivingssris.com). I have tried to keep the focus of this book strictly on the strategies I brought to bear in my effort discontinue and have selectively included portions of my own story, which are recounted in fuller measure on the blog under the category "Wendy's Story."

This book is not intended to serve as or to replace medical advice. It is merely a narrative about my journey and recounts what worked for me. Please, always consult a healthcare professional before making the decision to discontinue your medication.

A technical note: All footnotes are found at the end of the chapter in which they are noted.

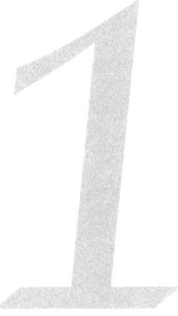

Take the Long View

Once you have resolved that the time has come to get off your medications, it is best to broach the process with the clear-headed reality that it is going to take some time. The idea of settling in for a long haul when it comes to getting off antidepressants can be a distressing prospect for anyone who is ready once and for all to be rid of these medications. This is a typical and normal response. We picture the heroic junkie tossing the drugs into the toilet, flushing, and then bracing for a few days of sweats and writhing. This is the wrong picture to envision when you have reached the place where you want to stop taking your antidepressants. First, you are not a junkie—you are someone whose brain has been chemically altered—and righting that alteration is going to take time and resolve. Second, there can be no flushing of these meds down the toilet. Reaching the place where you know it is time to stop is only the first step in what is destined to be a long road.

Consider how much preparation goes in to planning for a trip. Who will watch the dog? Who will water the plants? How will I pay for the extra costs? What kinds of clothing should I bring? Should I pack less in order to bring home more? The lists and contingencies are endless and one must ever be needing to grab a notepad and write down that one more item that needs to be accomplished before closing the door and walking away. Vacations often take months to plan for and may last only a few weeks. Discontinuation demands equal planning and may well last many months, if not years. In a way, I hope you will consider this book your "notepad" for preparation.

Several years ago, when I was writing my book on the life of Saint Francis of Assisi, I made the decision to move to Italy for the period of time it would take me to complete the book. The preparations for this move were daunting and felt untenable. The first step involved selling most of my possessions—except the really important ones—because I had no idea how long I would be gone and had no leeway to place my things in paid storage. Because I did not have the emotional reserves to price each and every item in my home, I simply opened cupboards and gave access to my rooms, cordoning off those specific corners of my little home where sniffers and buyers would have no entrance. Then, I left it to the shoppers to make me an offer on my things. It saved a lot of inner turmoil and time and for the most part the prices they bid were reasonable. That was one step. Then I had to spend three months before my departure living on the estate of a wealthy local resident, serving her cleaning person, personal assistant, cook and grocery shopper, again in anticipation of the move. I did not enjoy being in this position but I needed to make sufficient money to live on while I was in residence and writing overseas. Then there was the matter of updating the passport, taking Italian lessons, securing a living situation in Italy, deciding what to do with my car and packing the few items retained from the name-your-own-price house sale to take along with me. I packed 21 boxes, called an international shipper, and watched him carry away the last vestiges of my life within a few weeks of my departure, hoping blindly that these boxes would indeed arrive at my new locale once I was ensconced in my apartment in Assisi. (They did.)

This move took me six months of preparation. Then, once in Italy I lived there for the next 15 months. Before I knew it, I was back in the U.S. with little in the way of possessions and needing to start over again, but at least I had my book. (You can purchase it on Amazon.) The point being, I understood what needed to be done in order to write the book I had been contracted to write. I did whatever it took.

This mindset is a little bit like what needs to be brought to bear before beginning the journey of discontinuation. For the effort this will require, you need to resolve to do whatever it takes and to realize that for this season the primary mandate of your life is to help yourself get off the meds and to heal yourself.

Another way of looking at it is as if you were going into combat. You don't simply lurch forward swords bandied and arms flailing. The preparation for combat, all that the moment demands and will be brought to bear to secure victory, resides beneath the surface against the backdrop of your training. The same is true of discontinuation. You cannot succeed without the proper preparation and orientation. But when you establish yourself and prepare yourself to begin the journey, with time and patience, you will prevail. Your body will begin to adjust, slowly – achingly. But bodies are made to heal. That's what they do.

It is the brain we are talking about here. Give it the time it is going to need. Be patient. Set your face like flint. Make your preparations.

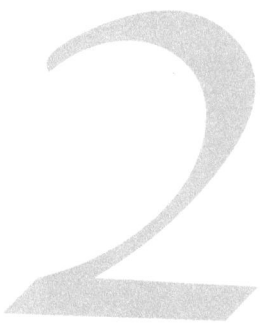

Determine Your Time

Once you have made the decision that the time has come to begin to taper and have resolved to do whatever it takes for as long as it takes, it is time to execute a plan. Several factors must be considered as you begin to plot out your "schedule" for tapering.

Bearing in mind that you will be diminishing your dosage by approximately 10 percent increments about every two to four weeks, you will quickly realize that if you start your taper at, say, 50 milligrams of whatever drug you are taking, getting down to zero at that rate will prove daunting. Some evidence suggests that a taper from higher milligram levels to a less-high milligram level isn't as jarring as tapering those last 10 milligrams. Studies similarly show that higher doses are no more effective than less-high dose, and in fact increase the chances of adverse side effects.[1]

For example, during my first attempt, my initial taper went from 40mg of citalopram to 20mg without a thought. I was doing the taper all wrong, not having researched it at that point, and I did experience some turmoil during that adjustment period. But at the time I did not attribute the struggle to the taper; other factors also made that particular stretch of my life difficult and I simply concluded I was experiencing a few bad days. Once that stretch settled out—and even after that disastrous first attempt required reinstatement—I never went back to that higher dosage.

All this to say, whatever reduction rate you appropriate, you may be able to reduce higher dosages a little more apace than those excruciating lower doses. Be sure to consult a supportive healthcare professional before beginning your taper. Once you have reached approximately 25mg, the real struggles begin. At this point you can anticipate minimally nine months or more before realizing complete and sustained discontinuation.

Season on the Calendar

The reason anticipating the timing is important is so that you can organize your withdrawal journey against a multiplicity of factors based on the time of year. When I began my third (and final) attempt, I had reached the point where I understood how rough the ride was going to be and in the effort to remove any unnecessary elements that could derail me, I planned based upon the calendar.

I started the taper in early May because this meant for the majority of it, the weather would make it possible to be outside and active. I am a gardener and derive great pleasure from being outside, planting, digging, pruning, transplanting – basically, doing all those small things that healthy gardens require to flourish. So I plotted the roughest patches of my taper around the months when I would be undertaking an activity that brought me pleasure and got me outside.

In addition to feeding the pleasure endorphins, the warmer weather also made it possible to consistently exert myself physically, which is an extremely valuable element of a successful taper. Physical activity keeps your blood circulating and the more blood that rushes through your brain, the better you will feel. Plus, your body will benefit from being physically expended and you will sleep better. Difficultly sleeping is a signature feature of tapering and everything you can do to help overthrow it will help you over the long haul.

Season of Life

Another important element to consider is the circumstance of your life at the time you begin a taper. During my first attempt, which failed, I was living in a place that was not working for me: I was far from my grown sons in a state and city where I knew very few people and was struggling to get work and to fit in. I was unhappy, in other words.

I rectified this situation before beginning a second taper. I moved back to the locale closer to my children –

thus removing one of the key obstacles that had proven a significant factor in my struggles. This was a good decision. Even so, the circumstances of my life even at that point were still a challenge and I discovered, this too, contributed to the sabotage of my second failed attempt to discontinue. Because I was financially compromised at the time of my move, I could afford only a room-rental arrangement. So whereas the move eliminated one of the primary factors that had so unsettled me during the first taper, it created another difficult feature that contributed to the turmoil of the second taper. The room rental arrangement was beneficial in many ways, but it was also constricting. I had no home to entertain in; I had no kitchen in which to share a family meal; no place to go other than "my room" when I was between other obligations.

There were many difficult trials with this second attempt, which I go into in the blog, and in the end I again reinstated – and my medication changed. I was destined for another several months of "readjustment" to the new medication and the additional pharmaceuticals one is obliged to take to keep the adjustment phase in check.

I waited several more months before starting to taper again. By that point I had moved into a more manageable living arrangement in a town where I already had a network of friends and colleagues. This was the point at which I made very clear calculations about the "season" of my life and whether or not the outer circumstances would support or sabotage my struggle.

I had determined, after great pains and a few misfires, that this was the time. Also at this point I had pretty much determined that this would be a do-or-die effort. I marked the day on the calendar and began, once again, the process of cutting tablets and keeping a log of my dosage.

1. See the following articles: "Dose-response relationship of recent antidepressants in the short-term treatment of depression," *Dialogues Clin Neurosci.* 2005 September; 7(3): 249–262, http://pubmedcentral-canada.ca/pmcc/articles/PMC3181733/; "Finding the 'Minimal Effective Dose' of Antidepressants & Other Drugs," *Mental Health Daily*, http://mentalhealthdaily.com/2015/01/16/finding-the-minimal-effective-dose-of-antidepressants-other-drugs/. See also a helpful blog post: "Does Antidepressant Dose Matter?" Kaz Thomas, http://asserttrue.blogspot.com/2013/04/dose-antidepressant-dose-matter.html.

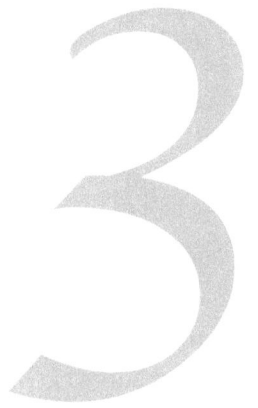

Choose Your Plan

Now you have come to the place where you are ready to plant your flag on a specific day on the calendar to begin to taper. By this point you will have made the determination 1) that the time has come to stop the meds; 2) that you are prepared to do whatever it takes to help yourself succeed at what is destined to be a long road; and 3) you have organized your life so that you can make this effort the foremost priority in the coming days.

By "choosing a plan" I mean putting together a concrete strategy. This begins with a starting point, but resist the temptation to set a deadline, that is, a pre-established time frame in which you hope to realize this goal. As you plan, it is best to do away with thoughts of deadlines. The primary concern during your taper is to preserve a degree of a quality of life while slowly, incrementally reducing your dosage. If your quality of life suffers in deference to a deadline, you are destined to fail and will inevitably need to reinstate at some point in order to regain minimal functionality. Try very hard not to set yourself up for this by not putting a deadline on this process.

Pick a Starting Date

Choose a beginning date that ideally falls at the start of a swathe of time wherein you have assurances of other things to do, particularly (if possible) the ability to be outside and active and in the sunshine. Early spring is a good time to start (if you live in a climate that has four seasons), since you can anticipate several months of temperate weather and the possibility of hikes or gardening or beach walks or sitting in the sun. All of these subtle recreational diversions are settling and life-giving during the process of tapering and the process is taken on day-by-day.

Prepare a List of Things to Do

As part of your plan make a list of activities you can undertake during the harder moments. Keep that list ever before your mind because, inevitably, what will happen during the disequilibrium of the taper is that your thinking will become confused, you will become agitated, distracted and distraught. If you have a pre-written list of "things to do" during one of these difficult moments—and then follow it—you will find you can get through another day. The battle to get off these meds is one wherein ground is taken by the inch. So help yourself ahead of time by preparing a contingency plan for something to do when the demon rears its head and you feel like you are losing your way. (See a sample list in the Addenda at the back of the book.)

Determine Your Sequence of Dose Reduction

The generally accepted sequence of reduction is in 10 percent increments. That means that if you are settled in at 25mg, you will begin your taper by taking 22.5mg (10 percent of 25 is 2.5; 25 - 2.5 = 22.5). As you begin you will need to monitor yourself and keep track of what symptoms may come upon you. Chances are, you will feel some agitation and restlessness, maybe some intense anger. But at this slow decrease in dosage, these symptoms will be both anticipated and manageable. When you begin to feel them you will know what they are and can then consult your predetermined list of things to do and go do something. These symptoms, at a 10-percent taper, may last for a few weeks but at some point you will begin to feel them subside. Once they subside, wait another week. Once you've navigated approximately two weeks of minimal—or no—symptoms, you can then drop down another 10 percent. Again, using the example above: if you have been taking 22.5mg you will drop to 20.25mg. This process will continue for many months during which time, day-by-day, it will help you to track your symptoms and appropriate activities you've noted on your list. Over time, these notations will bring you encouragement about your progress.

A word about tapering: Doctors themselves often tell their patients who want to taper simply to start halving their doses. This where the unique chemistry of varying individuals must be intuited and determined by each person. Generally, it is thought that it is easier to go from—say 40mg to 20mg of Celexa than it is to go from 10mg to 0mg. As already mentioned, high doses to less-high dose may be able to be realized at increments greater than 10 percent. Consult your healthcare professional and, if you do a drop early on that is higher than 10 percent, monitor yourself closely and, if need be, reinstate at a lesser dose, let yourself settle out, then resume the taper more gradually. Only you know your own body. Consult your healthcare professional before beginning the taper, but always remember that only you can feel what is happening inside you.

As for how to lessen your dose, there are a couple of ways you can go about it. I know one man who systematically shaved literally dust-amounts off his pills with a nail file. He would track his reductions by the number of swipes: for each taper reduction he would add another two swipes of the file. Others (including myself) have asked their doctors to give them a prescription for a liquid version of their medication and then would measure each taper by lines on the syringe. Still others (again, myself among them during my third attempt) have simply used the tried-and-true method of pill slicing. None of these is a perfect technique, but each of them does push the process forward. The key to whatever method you choose is to always be monitoring your symptoms.

Your body will tell you if the drop has been too much. You must find that thin line between succumbing to the agitation and pressing on, giving your brain the needed time to adjust. A good basic rule of thumb is, if you are feeling difficult symptoms, give yourself a few weeks. If they persist beyond that point, think about tapering at a slower rate. It is always a delicate dance. Every day you are taking stock of how you feel and if your are able to manage the disequilibrium your taper is imposing.

A final word: each person's taper is as unique as that person's brain chemistry. During my taper, when I consulted others about my regimen, one person in particular who had researched the science behind tapering thoroughly and shepherded many people through this process, registered concern to me about certain aspects of my taper. I appreciated her concern but the effect her lecturing had on me was to throw me into confusion and distress amid an already delicate process. In truth, my taper was going well; it was working. After considering her concerns, in the end I dismissed them because only I knew what was going on inside my system and I knew that what I was doing was working. I was not going to disrupt this because someone else deemed my strategy flawed. All that to say, you will receive a lot of advice. Some of it will be extremely helpful and some of it will bring you down. Keep your feet firmly planted in your strategy and, as long as you are monitoring yourself, being wise, circumspect and vigilant—keep the course you have set and don't allow the opinions of others to throw confusion in your process.

4

Batten Down the Hatches

If this chapter title sounds dramatic, it is intended to. The storms that rage inside your mind during the process of discontinuation are tumultuous and unless you are ready for them—they will defeat you when they come in all their fury. On my blog I wrote about the storms of the taper this way:

> *"[You] feel by turns the bitter change*
> *Of fierce extremes, extremes more fierce*
> *From beds of raging fire to starve in ice*
> *Their soft ethereal warmth, and there to pine*
> *Immovable, infixed, and frozen round,*
> *Periods of time . . .*
>
> *"No rest; through many a dark and dreary vale*
> *They passed, and many a region dolorous,*

Wendy Murray

O'er many a froze, many a fiery Alp,
Rocks, caves, lakes, fens, bogs, dens,
and shades of death,
A universe of death . . .

John Milton, *Paradise Lost*

This passage from Milton captures the picture of my struggle to get off antidepressants. It was a long, tedious slog that summoned every ounce of human grit from every corner of my physical, emotional and spiritual apparatus. I have learned that it is also the picture of millions of other strugglers' efforts to get off these drugs. We are hidden band fighting epic battles inside our minds even as we do the laundry, check out books from the library or show up to work.

This is because something in the brain of a person who is discontinuing sends alarming signals. Often these impulses leave one with the singular feeling of rage that focuses on the need to self-destruct or to destroy something or someone else.

For those who are discontinuing, even if they do manage not to act upon these impulses, there will be many more battles to come which may or may not yield another inch. All the while the intractable rage impulse ravages the mind – "rocks, caves, lakes, fens, bogs, dens, and shades of death, a universe of death"– while you are checking out books from the library, doing laundry, or showing up for work.

That is why I say "batten down the hatches." The

storm will come. It will be hard and you will doubt yourself. In fact, you may hate yourself and heap all manner of abuse upon yourself. Consult your list at this point. Self-loathing is one of most toxic and deceitful elements of what happens to your mind while you are tapering. Amid all the chemically-induced piston-firing going on inside one's brain is the specter of self-rebuke, self-diminishment, self-reproach—self, self, self. You hear yourself say, What have you accomplished? Who, in the world, needs you? These are lies, but they pound steadily. They are inside your head speaking more force- fully than the whispers of angels. In every way you are able, try to step outside yourself during these periods and help yourself by talking down these lies. You are a sailor in a storm trying to save the ship.

What SSRIs Do

The key to understanding why these symptoms show themselves as they do lies in the chemical manipula- tions caused in the brain when a person is taking an SSRI.

The term itself—'Selective Serotonin Re-uptake Inhibi- tors'—is a roundabout way of saying these drugs inhibit the natural recycling of serotonin. In simpler terms, it is helpful to think of SSRIs as running defense on the natu- ral cyclical flow of serotonin between nerve endings.

In a normal nervous system serotonin in the brain is sent from the "sending" nerve ending to a "receiving" nerve ending. The locus of this exchange is the syn- apse—the no-man's land that exists between sending and receiving nerves. The "Sender" releases serotonin which enters the synapse, there to be absorbed into the nerve ending of the "Receiver." Whatever serotonin is not absorbed by the Receiver gets flushed back into the Sender to be recycled and eventually re-released, making for a lively give-and-take between the Sender and the Receiver. When SSRIs are introduced they change the terms of this dance. The Senders still send and the Receivers still receive. But those random bits of serotonin that don't get initially absorbed are blocked from being recycled into the Senders and forced back into the Receiver, thus the denotation "selected serotonin re-uptake inhibitor."

SSRIs increase serotonin in the brain by forcing molecules back into the Receiving nerve ending that otherwise should have been reabsorbed by the Sending nerve ending. As a result, the brain is experiencing more serotonin impulses on the Receiving nerve, which enables the patient to feel better for a while. But this effect is temporary. When the drug is preventing the serotonin from being recycled, it means two things. First, for a time, the Receiver is over-stimulated by forced serotonin, while, second, the Sender is gradually becoming depleted because of the lack of recycling. The serotonin becomes deficient in the Sender, which begins to short circuit some of the Receivers waiting to receive. SSRIs sabotage the natural recycling effect between nerves, altering the connection between the Sending / Receiving neurons at the synapse, disabling the re-uptake pump (a pore) that flushes the serotonin back into the

Sender to be recycled.

This re-uptake-inhibiting process that SSRIs use to increase serotonin levels in the brain is at the heart of the withdrawal problem. By blocking serotonin receptors on Sending neurons, the natural send-receive synergy has been interrupted, and as a result the brain becomes chemically dependent upon the drug to maintain consistent levels of serotonin. As the brain becomes accustomed to the drug, it no longer resorts to its normal function of producing or regulating serotonin and no longer functions with the normal cycle of sending, receiving and recycling of serotonin. During the process of tapering, as the SSRI chemical is removed from the now-altered brain, the levels of serotonin fluctuate in the neurotransmitters. The system gets gummed up and the brain isn't firing on all pistons, the way an engine in a car would get gummed if some sabotaging agent were thrown into its pistons. This fluctuation causes wide mood swings and uncontrollable emotions, as evidenced in the struggles of the thousands of people on forum web sites.

The brain is trying to adjust to the need to self-regulate levels of serotonin. In the meantime many patients, myself among them, experience a cascade of extreme emotional and physical symptoms that include debilitating depression, anxiety, panic, rage, confusion, agitation, crying spells, insomnia, memory loss, general aches, headaches and heart palpitations. These symptoms can feel quite unmanageable and so intense that you become hopeless in the face of them and see no way out. The electrical impulses in the brain are going haywire and the result is that the standard mechanism used to control emotions is no longer functioning appropriately. Withdrawal triggers the mind to respond more viscerally and in a way completely disconnected from normal thought processes and standard restraints. In a normally functioning brain, cognition regulates visceral responses moderating in proportion to the circumstances that aroused them. SSRI withdrawal disconnects the mind from this regulatory function so that moderating behavior is overthrown by unmanageable emotional impulses of anger, fear, and anxiety. Anger normally can be managed. For example, when someone cuts you off while driving you may call them an idiot but you won't pull out a gun and shoot them. Withdrawal removes that moderating behavior and allows rage to become the singular dominant and irrational response, which—in the case of the driver who cuts you off—might explain certain incidents of "road rage." Uncontrollable rage springs fully formed in the mind and propels itself toward an unsuspecting target, as if an external force has hijacked that person's personality, as indeed it has. Other emotional symptoms of withdrawal act in a similar way – inexplicable crying fits, overwhelming panic. Even for the patient who exercises mindful self-awareness, these symptoms come on with little warning causing great turbulence and possess a visceral realness that most people find alarming. The brain's chemical balance has been disrupted, so reality itself for the patient has been altered. Instead of an emotional wave that must be conquered or endured, these emotions become reality itself, with a feeling of inevitability that sometimes ends in tragedy.

During some of the worst periods of this disequilibrium while I was suffering I consulted a very helpful blog hosted by a man named James. James had an articulate and helpful way of explaining what was happening during these storms and it enabled me and many readers of his blog to help navigate them. He has given me permission to reproduce portions of his blog posts here.

James explained these emotional torrents as experiencing "wave" and "windows":

One of the frustrating parts of withdrawal is the way that symptoms fluctuate over time. People call them waves and windows. At first, withdrawal is unremitting and there seems to be no respite from the symptoms. After some time, which varies from person to person, symptoms begin to break up into cycles. There are times when symptoms aren't as bad, and other times when they are quite severe, which I call the wave/window pattern. It's not a universal pattern, but it seems to be true in the majority of cases.

Waves
Waves describe those times when symptoms are more severe. Symptoms can be physical or emotional. It feels like getting sick. When you start to get a cold, you can feel little changes that presage

the illness. A sore throat or headache, then the full symptoms of the cold start in a day or two. A wave has similar precursors. Usually, physical symptoms are the first sign that a wave is coming. A stiff neck, headaches, and dizziness are some of the symptoms. A day or two later, the emotional symptoms become more pronounced. These symptoms include obsessive or compulsive thoughts, depression, or anxiety. It can be helpful to break waves up into different parts. Knowing that each part of a wave is coming, and what to expect next, can make the whole process easier to handle. The reason we're so adept at knowing the cycle of a cold is that we've had them off and on all our lives. We're aware of the subtle changes in our bodies that tell us that we're getting sick. In the same way, it takes some experience before you can separate the parts of a wave from each other. It takes still more time to develop ways of dealing with each part of a wave.

Physical symptoms of a wave are hard to mitigate. There isn't much you can do about general joint pain, headaches, or dizziness. You can try analgesics like aspirin or ibuprofen, but those aches are fairly resistant to those kinds of pain killers. Dizziness is likewise difficult to deal with. Withdrawal dizziness isn't just something that happens when you stand up or spin around. It's hard to believe that you can feel dizzy when you lie down, but it happens in withdrawal. Try to stay as still as possible until it gets better. Try to use the physical symptoms as a sign that there are new symptoms coming that you need to deal with.

There isn't really any way to avoid the emotional symptoms of a wave. There is no way to "suck it up and get over it." The anxiety, depression, and obsessions of a wave are just as real as the screen in front of you. The fact that our rational mind would recognize that it's not real or overblown doesn't mean much when you're experiencing it. That's the essence of a wave. It's not rational. Obsessive thoughts can be about almost anything from the benign to the surreal. Self harm can suddenly seem like a rational plan.

In normal thought, the entire spectrum of emotions are right below the surface. In withdrawal, thoughts that would normally be dismissed gain the same weight in our conscious minds as socially acceptable thoughts. The only way to mitigate the emotional symptoms of a wave is to be mindful of the difference between normal thought and the unnatural power of irrational thought that occurs in a wave. It's very hard to pick apart which thoughts are your normal responses and which ones are caused by the wave. They mingle together in a chaotic way. That's what makes your reactions to a window just as important as your reactions to a wave.

Windows

Windows are those periods of time when symptoms are not as pronounced. At first a window might even fool you into thinking you've beat withdrawal, you're free. That's the cruel joke of SSRI withdrawal. Windows and waves are intertwined together. The way withdrawal works for most people is that the windows slowly, ever so slowly, get longer, and the waves get shorter. A window is more than a vacation from symptoms. It is a huge relief to have some time off from feeling miserable. Savor the good times in withdrawal, because that is what you have to look forward to in recovery. More than relief, though, windows are an opportunity to prepare yourself to deal with waves in a better way. Try to pay attention to how you feel. Examine the way you think, the way you respond to things. Try to recognize the way that you automatically choose responses and thoughts. Emotionally, a window is a return to the normal way of parsing thoughts. Paying attention to the thought processes during a window makes it easier to impose that same kind of structure during the next wave. It's that mindfulness that you'll need during the next wave. After a while, you can tell when a thought is out of character and consciously dismiss it.

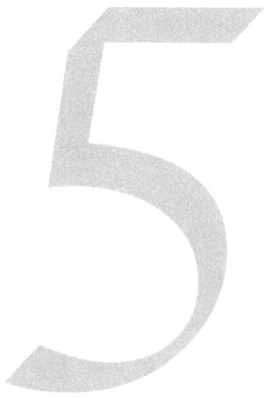

Anticipate Distress

The most debilitating aspect of enduring a taper is the battle that unfolds inside your mind. If you are on antidepressants in the first place then someone concluded that you were emotionally compromised enough to warrant chemical intervention. This will be one point of attack that will rear its head during the long and troubled hidden moments of your taper.

I have pondered why, when tapering, the symptoms take on the aspect of an intensified, unrelenting mental assault – why not, say, euphoria? How pleasant would it be if, during the time of readjustment our brains instead went haywire into the realm of unharnessed ecstasy! As it is, we are left debilitated and laid low by unharnessed rage, sorrow, panic or despair. The challenge of the taper first, is to recognize these emotional extremes for what they are: chemical adjustments, and, second, to cultivate habits to keep them in check.

In the midst of it, it is almost impossible to take stock of what is happening. And even if you are able, taking stock does not necessarily translate into the ability to cope. You are being assaulted on several fronts: psychological, emotional and physical. I mention the latter because, as much as any other aspect of this journey, the physical symptoms will feed into the emotional turmoil you are experiencing.

Among the most daunting physical side effect is insomnia, a signature feature of discontinuation. It also carries the potential to derail the whole project. It is during the long hours of insomnia where (it feels like it anyway) the battle is won or lost. During my third taper I had begun a regimen of herbal tinctures to try and help my body compensate for the lessening chemicals (this will be discussed in more detail later). Attempting to avert insomnia, cleanse my system, and achieve a degree of equilibrium, I would take tinctures during the day. Then, as evening would fall, I would take tinctures to settle my raving system in the attempt to achieve repose. And there were some nights when the drift of sleep would fall over me and I counted these occasions blessed. Yet as I reached lower milligrams the tinctures didn't cut it and I would find myself making justifications for why it was necessary to take other chemicals simply to induce sleep. I would exist in this bizarre symbiosis of purity and balance by way of tinctures during the day and ravings and desperation in the night. One of my physicians who helped me during the third attempt told me if I was having too much trouble sleeping that she would write me a prescription for Trazadone. She said that my taper will not succeed if I don't sleep ("sleep deprivation is a form of torture," she said). I never took her up on the offer not wanting yet another chemical to be thrown into the mix. I already had in my possession some leftover meds from previous tapers. So during the difficult long, desperate hours of sleeplessness that I knew would translate into lethargy, hopelessness and incapacitation when morning came, there were concessions that had to be made. I would take a sleeping aid. It will feel like a vicious cycle: taking Ambien to come off citalopram; taking diazepam to come off Ambien. This was a battle I knew would not be resolved that night. This is the kind of moment when you gather yourself and remind yourself that your singular primary goal in this moment is to help yourself get off your antidepressant. There will be many more battles on many fronts. But you cannot fight every battle on the varied fronts all at once. Fight one battle on this singular front and bend everything you do to taking ground in that battle. So, if you find yourself raving in your bed unable to sleep and dreading the long hours until the sun comes up and you find you must face a day with nothing in your tank, do what you need to do to eliminate that battle. Take a pill. You will not feel good about it. And you may not feel well, physically or emotionally, when you arise in the morning. But the key here is that you arise, that is, from sleep. You will not succeed if you don't sleep.

There will be a day and another battle to be fought

when it comes to diminishing your sleep medication. And, over time, as your body recovers you will find you have the physical reserves to take on that battle.

At the intense stages of antidepressant discontinuation you must continuously remind yourself that getting off this med is your one and only goal. Bend everything you do that goal. If going out with friends inevitably derails your momentum, throwing off your sleeping or otherwise exacerbating your emotions, then don't go out with your friends. Be your own friend. Help yourself get through this. Your friends will understand. If they don't then they are not your friends.

Be Patient

During the long hours of reckoning and reclaiming my mind and spirit while discontinuing, I found myself drawn to the writings of a group of religious ascetics known as the "Desert Fathers." They were a small band of religious monks who had renounced the world, wealth, and earthly consolation to live in the desert of Egypt around the third century A.D. They eschewed all pleasures of the senses, rich food, baths, leisure, and anything luxurious in deference to a life of poverty, simplicity, chastity and prayer.

I am not sure what drew me to their writings during this time, but long ago I stopped trying to justify various tools or habits I found helpful to get me through my tapering. I suppose it might have been due, in part, to the fact that the Desert Fathers lived more or less inside their minds and spirits, spending all their time praying, meditating, singing psalms, fasting – all while trying to preserve harmony with one another and keeping their thoughts and desires for God alone. It was an extreme expression of Christian devotion that arose in the aftermath of great persecution of Christians by the Roman Emperor Diocletian in 303 A.D.

I read about a novice who seemed nonplused about how these monks spent their time, since all their efforts went toward interior work. He asked an aged father, "What do you do all day?" The father answered, "Fall down and then pick myself up." His point was that the battles he confronted inside his head were unrelenting and required ongoing vigilance, patience, and self-forgiveness.

The power and simplicity of this monk's answer attests how even great men of God fought many battles inside their minds and sometimes fell down. In some ways the fierce interior struggles of the person who is tapering can be likened to this. Feelings of failure and sometimes even assault can overwhelm the person who is tapering and there is a temptation to allow these destructive feelings to upset the progress of the future course. At moments such as this, it is imperative to access your helpful self and rise up and hear yourself say (as the elderly monk did), "I have fallen down; now I must pick myself up."

There will be many moments when you will feel all is hopeless; that you are incapable of succeeding; that your body is too compromised to ever recover from this. Insofar as you are able, speak peace to yourself in these moments. The Scottish sailor, Andrew Barton, was a High Admiral of the Kingdom of Scotland of whom it was written in an early ballad:

> *I am hurt but I am not slain.*
> *I'll lay me down and bleed awhile*
> *then I'll rise and fight again.*

If need be, attend to yourself as the wounded warrior, take time to bleed. Then pick yourself up, put on your boots. There are more battles to be fought. Take your time. Help yourself get through them. Be patient. But get back up.

7

Record Your Dosage Reduction

By my third attempt to quit these meds I had figured out the routine: mark on the calendar the day your taper began; indicate the dose you've reduced to; keep track of how you are feeling day to day. This means having a calendar or appointment book or some other means to keep a log, which you will find yourself consulting more often than you may have originally anticipated.

For example, the point at which I began my second taper I had leveled out at 10mg of Celexa and determined to do a 10 percent taper. So, on a Thursday, I wrote "Started a 10% taper today/9mg." On Friday I wrote "9mg/2.5mg" – the 2.5 indicating that I had taken 2.5mg of Ambien the night before to help me sleep. Six weeks later, sensing that my body had adjusted, I wrote, again on a Thursday: "Began another 10% taper, down to 8.1." On day 5 after this drop I wrote (Tuesday): "Agitation." For the subsequent eight days, my calendar entries read as follows: (Wednesday): "Felt very out of sorts"; (Thursday) "Out of sorts"; (Friday): "Out of Sorts"; (Saturday): "Felt awful in the a.m. but improved greatly"; (Sunday): "Felt very bound up / sad / broken / in pain"; (Monday): "Felt a little relief"; (Tuesday): "Felt a little relief"; (Wednesday): "Felt better today"; and so on. It was four and a half weeks before I dropped another 10 percent—now to 7.2mg and I continued day by day to monitor how I felt. Again, on the fifth day after the drop I wrote in the calendar: "Started to feel effects of the taper; pounding heart, some depression." Two days later: "Felt intensity / heart pounding."

The struggles of the taper happen day to day and on any given day you can experience any number of symptoms. Then, on some days, you will feel relief. By documenting of all of this, over time, you to begin to see a pattern as to how your body is reacting to the drop in medication. Once you understand that—as in my case —the difficult symptoms begin to show themselves around day five, then you can manage them better and even plan accordingly. In my case, with each drop, these difficult symptoms lasted in force for approximately two weeks (beginning about on day five). That meant, for me, my body needed, minimally, about four weeks to adjust before I would drop again.

In addition to monitoring day by day what my dose was and how I was feeling, I had written elsewhere a taper schedule so that I could anticipate the pacing. Since my starting point had been 10mg the taper schedule looked like this:

9.00mg ⇨ 8.10 ⇨ 7.20 ⇨ 6.50 ⇨ 5.85 ⇨ 5.27 ⇨ 4.70 ⇨ 4.20 ⇨ 3.78 ⇨ 3.40 ⇨ 3.00 ⇨ 2.78 ⇨ 2.50 ⇨ 2.24 ⇨ 2.00 ⇨ 1.81 ⇨ 1.60 ⇨ 1.50 ⇨ 1.31 ⇨ 1.20 ⇨ 1.00 ⇨ .96 ⇨ .87 ⇨ .78 ⇨ .70

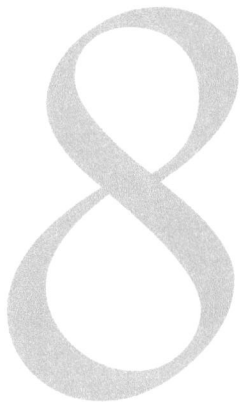

Track Your Emotions

This relentless recording of my days proved at once helpful and distressing during my second attempt. The tapers had been manageable, though not easy. As noted, my calendar entries included notations such as "fatigued / heart pounding" and "Felt off all day / anxiety." These kinds of entries fell under the taper that marked the 7.2mg stage. The most alarming aspect of this stage of the taper was the seemingly unrelenting heart pounding. There were times I was sure it would burst from the pressure. Vigorous walking helped this somewhat—but there were days when I felt so exhausted I could not bring myself to walk. But it was after my drop to 6.5mg that my symptoms deteriorated notably. (I determined this only by looking at my calendar log where I saw clearly a new and troubling pattern.) By day two at 6.5mg I wrote "Some weirdness / mild 'zapping."

Day 3: "a little head weirdness"

Day 4: "heart pounding / hysterical laughing"

Day 5: "Headache"

Day 6: "Headache / dull aching / no strength"

Day 7: "Dull headache / minor agitation / anxiety

Day 8: "Dull headache / Some achiness – Sleeplessness

Day 9: "Ongoing dull headache / great fatigue

Day 10: "Dizziness / head disequilibrium / very fatigued / headache / despair (I will never overcome my circumstances)"

Day 11: "Sleeplessness / no headache / fatigue lessened"

Day 12: "Some headaching / less fatigued"

Day 13: "Anxiety / dark thoughts / darkness"

Day 14: "Felt definitive darkness / struggle"

Day 15: "Morosely depressed / very tired"

Day 16: "One stretch of extreme anxiety, then settled"

Day 17: "Some anxiety re $ / 1/2 valium later 1/2 ativan"

Day 18: "Sorrow / missing my father / loneliness"

Day 19: "Felt okay / no crushing darkness"

Day 20: "Some darkness" . . .

The fact that for three solid weeks after I had tapered to 6.5mg I experienced unrelenting difficulties began to alarm me. Still I persisted. I did not drop my dosage—clearly my body had not yet adjusted—nor did I give up. I held steady at 6.5mg and continued to monitor how I felt. These harrowing symptoms at the 6.5mg-stage of my taper persisted for four weeks and were not improving, but alas were deteriorating. I took the initiative to see someone who I had been told, specialized in helping patients navigate the rough stages of tapering, which proved to be quite the opposite, actually. This health-care professional promptly changed my medication and reinstated me at 25mg of Zoloft.

My point is, my relentless tracking of emotions and symptom enabled me to take a step back and see, objectively, that the taper was not going well and that I needed to do something. Sometimes this effort can be circuitous; sometimes it is necessary to back track in order to get right and straight-sighted before going on.

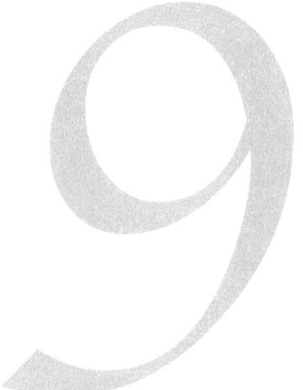

Eat Healthily

A critical element to helping your body make the needed transition to health and wholeness resulting from the debilitating effects of SSRIs is physical functionality. It is very difficult to overcome the struggle to get off the meds if your body is fighting other battles.

Before you begin your taper take stock of your general health and do what you can to help your body prepare for the long journey getting off meds. Even so, avoid the temptation to diet with the hope of becoming svelte and sleek. Set reasonable goals and bend your will to achieve healthy choices.

Chances are you may have put on some pounds as a result of the medication. I never had a problem with weight until I was put on Zoloft, at which point I ballooned. I desperately wanted to lose that extra weight, even as I was trying to get off the Zoloft. But in the end

I deferred to getting off Zoloft and didn't count calories. That said, the calories I did consume were of a kind that would only help my body function better. For example, some well-known weight loss establishments warn people off of fats such as are found in avocado and olive oil. Yet both avocados and olive oil are excellent sources of oleic acid, a monounsaturated fatty acid that is believed to be "heart-healthy." When it comes to foods such as these, ignore the calorie count and help your heart beat more vigorously and efficiently and your blood to flow stronger.

Do what you can to stop eating "processed foods." Many of the staples of the average diet contain processed foods, which means simply that the stuff you are putting in your mouth has been altered in some way from its original state. In some instances this processing does not hurt the food – for example, freezing fruit and vegetables preserves nutrients during long-term storage.

Unfortunately, the processing in much of today's food products goes way beyond this necessity. Ingredients such as salt, sugar and fat are sometimes added to processed foods to make their flavor more appealing and to prolong their shelf life. Highly processed foods tend to be less digestible, with lower absorption in the body and often higher in calories. In other words, your body has to work harder to derive any nutritional benefit and often the nutrients are lacking. These foods also tend to be higher in "bad calories," unlike the avocado, which is filled with good calories.

Remember: The purpose of improving your diet is not to lose weight or to look better. It is to help your body function at its optimal efficiency because a healthy heart and well-flowing blood is going to be needed to counter the assault that diminishing your meds will inflict.

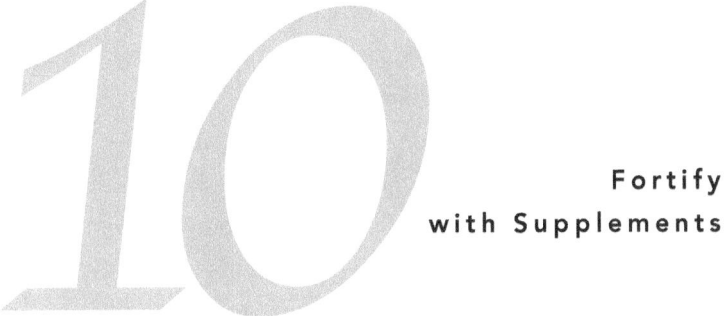

Fortify
with Supplements

Before launching into a discussion about supplements it is important to clarify that I do not consider myself a nutritionist, dietician or an herbalist. The information I include in this chapter is derived from my personal experience with supplements and the associated research I undertook, highlighting what worked for me. This section is intended to offer a beginning point to grasp the value of supplements in aiding the journey to successful tapering and to point you in the direction so that you can undertake your own research and experimentation.

That said, anyone attempting to taper successfully needs to understand that dietary supplements are wonderful gifts that can make a significant difference in the success of your efforts. These gifts are derived directly from earth and organic chemistry and will go a long way in helping your body and your brain recover from the ravages of antidepressant use. Supplements include vitamins, minerals, herbs or other plants, and amino acids. They are widely available in health food stores, grocery stores, pharmacies, on the Internet, and by mail. You're probably aware of many supplements and may already be using them. Common ones include products such as St. John's wort, melatonin, Vitamin B complex, fish oils, essential oils, tinctures and the like.

Makers of dietary supplements cannot legally say that their products can diagnose, cure, treat, or prevent disease. The U.S. Food and Drug Administration (FDA) does not regulate dietary supplements in the same way that it regulates medicine. But they can say that supplements contribute to health maintenance and well-being.

People have used dietary supplements for thousands of years to help health and to treat illness. Sometimes those supplements are the basis for some of today's common medicines. For example, people have used willow bark tea for centuries to relieve fever and as a result pharmaceutical companies eventually identified the chemical in willow bark that relieved fever and used that knowledge to produce aspirin. Many of the medicines of modern science have been designed to imitate the benefits of medicines from nature. The chemical composition in Valium has tried to mimic the effects of Valerian root.

During my second taper I began taking (and cultivating) medicinal herbs and made tinctures, particularly from Valerian root and holy basil. I used these tinctures every day to help deal with the negative effects of the tapering. Through my experience with herbs and tinctures I have come to appreciate the value of these gifts of the earth which really do give us everything we need to maintain our health. The benefits of herbals are long-term but keep in mind, being herbs, the process takes more time than the typical "immediate relief" people commonly expect and receive from pharmaceuticals.

In this way treating yourself to herbs simultaneously with the taper is a proportional way to help keep your system in balance. The taper happens slowly in small incremental steps; herb and supplement healing also happens slowly and incrementally. So it's not too soon to begin!

Though my second attempt did not succeed, I did not abandon taking the tinctures and the supplements as I progressed. Even when I had to reinstate, I kept these healing life-giving benefits in my system so that when I began to taper again, this time for the third attempt, my body was much more fortified and healthy than any of the previous two times I had tried. I credit the supplements for this success, along with the aspects of body and mind (and soul) preparedness that I outline in this book.

You will not hear a lot from your doctor about supplements because, as one fellow successful taperer put it (who also works in the mental health industry), "docs don't get 'educated' by supplement companies the way they get 'educated' by pharmaceutical companies."

There needs to be a degree of forethought that goes

into how you are going to broach your taper and the supplements you may decide to take. It would be best to start with certain ones that are tried and true when it comes to general health and wellbeing.

Some of these include: holy basil (tea or tincture) that has wonderful calming attributes and a pleasant spicy taste; Valerian root (capsules or tincture), which is very effective in helping cope with insomnia; it also has calming attributes. Fish oil and omega 3-6-9 (fish, flax and borage oils) are very good for brain function.

As my third taper reached critical levels as I moved into lower milligrams—that pressure point where my first two attempts had failed—I introduced certain supplements that proved to be for me the decisive game-changer that got me through the final tortured milligrams and enabled me, at long last, to cross the finish line. These helped carry me through that critical hit-the-wall stage.

As I drew closer to the low milligram counts (at about 10 mg) I started taking tryosine and omega 3-6-9, to enhance cognitive function. When I got to 6mg I introduced L-tryptophan, also known as 5-HTP (5-hydroxy-tryptophan). 5-HTP is an amino acid made from extracts of the seeds of the African tree *Griffonia simplicifolia*. It is a chemical that the body makes from tryptophan (an essential amino acid that you get from food). After tryptophan is converted into 5-HTP, the chemical is changed into serotonin – you know what that is: the neurotransmitter that relays signals between brain cells; (see Chapter 4). 5-HTP dietary supplements helps raise serotonin levels in the brain, which helps off-set the trauma and disequilibrium associated with coming off of SSRIs. The supplement can help regulate mood and anxiety and also may have a positive effect on sleep. (See the appendix for more important information about this supplement.)

5-HTP proved to be especially helpful for me during the struggles of the low doses. Because it produces more serotonin it is important to hold off taking it until closer to the end of your taper. At that point it helped my brain get through the intense lowering of artificially-induced increased serotonin that occurs with SSRIs.

For a list of additional supplements see the Addenda.

Get Exercise

Getting out and moving is an important and incomparable must-have in order to succeed at tapering. I say "getting out" because so much of the battle of med reduction is fought inside one's head, that the very act of grabbing the keys to the car or putting on a sweatshirt for a vigorous walk changes your interior landscape and helps stave off anxiety and melt-downs.

Obviously, the most important benefit of exercise is the life-giving robust energy it brings to the heart and muscles, which in turn benefit the brain. When you exercise, your body releases chemicals called endorphins, which act as analgesics—pain reducers—interacting with the receptors in the brain that reduce your perception of pain. Endorphins also trigger a positive feeling in the body, which is why, for example, runners often describe their workouts as euphoric. Endorphins are manufactured in the brain, spinal cord, and many other parts of your body and are released in response to neurotransmitters in the brain. All of this works toward healing your brain during the difficult days of the taper.

In short, regular exercise is a critical element that will aid you in successfully tapering off antidepressants. Not only does the endorphin action reduce stress, diminish feelings of anxiety and depression, but you will also find that your sleep improves, the pounding of the heart relieved, and the fatigue not as overwhelming. Regular exercise also lowers blood pressure, improves muscle strength, strengthens bones and reduces body fat.

That said, don't go at a new exercise regimen with the thought that a month later you will have dropped two sizes. That is neither the point nor the goal of getting exercise. If it is, you will be disappointed, and disappointment is the enemy of success when it comes to the effective taper. If you are overweight, you are not going to solve that issue easily and trying to do so during the taper should not be your intent. (This is the same point noted in the section about diet.) Your intent is to get off the meds. If you should happen to reap the additional benefit of losing weight, then glory be. But stay focused on your singular purpose: to help yourself succeed, step-by-step, at getting off the antidepressants.

Depending upon your physical condition when you begin the taper, measure your physical regimen accordingly. The suggested minimum exercise plan is to walk for 30 minutes a day, three times a week, preferably at a level that elevates your heart rate to achieve a good pumping workout (an aerobic workout). If you can't reach or sustain this kind of output, simply do what you can. Do something, because anything is better than nothing. The more you get your blood flowing the better it will be for your brain specifically and your overall well-being generally.

At the gym I attend for my walks and work-outs I see many elderly and overweight people bringing their best effort to get around the walking track. I want to salute them. It cannot be easy and I see that often they must stop to catch their breath and simply recover from the exertion. But there they are, day by day and step by step, giving it an effort. One man in particular I have noticed who, when he started was morbidly overweight and, as the days and slow walks around the track have transitioned into months, I am seeing him have to pull his belt tighter around his diminishing waist. Good for him! No one laughs or ridicules him, though at first he lumbered and struggled to get around the track even a single time. We all in our hearts are cheering him on! And seeing his persistence and the diminishment of his waistline is a sight we rejoice in with him.

So if you are out of shape and cannot imagine yourself taking that first step, think again. The human body is an amazing thing and if you help it, you will find it will rise and grow strong and recover and render you gifts you thought may have been beyond your reach. To succeed at the taper, help your body. When you do that, you'll find your body will help you.

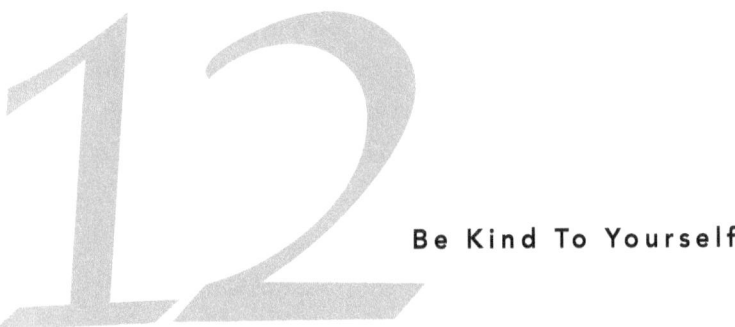

Be Kind To Yourself

During my journey to discontinuation I faced many, many moments when I felt utterly alone. While some in my closest circle knew I was tapering, in the darkest and hardest moments, when I did not know if I could survive this, there was no one in my life who walked side-by-side with me, whispering hopeful encouragement in my ear. While some knew of the tapering, no one stood guard over me or picked me up when I felt thrown down. That is not the case for others. I have read on many forums that some people would not have survived the journey without the support of a particular loved one who stood by them throughout.

My sense of it is this: rejoice if you get hands-on immediate support in this struggle, but don't assume it will be there. Be prepared to face the demons alone. In the end, with or without support, this is your battle and only you can take ground in it.

In this way it is very important that, throughout, you make an extra effort to be kind to yourself. Only you can help yourself and in this struggle there will be plenty of other negative forces trying to bring you down. You must not be one of those forces. You must be a positive force in your own journey, one of the forces that lifts you up. That is why, when you feel you are falling—or do, in fact, fall—be patient with yourself and like the Desert Father that I mentioned earlier, keep picking yourself up, even if it means doing it all day long. Sleep when you must sleep; stay home when you must stay home; go out when you must go out. Put a hedge of protection around yourself and do not let anyone broach it unless they are there to assist you unconditionally. Your only goal during this struggle is to help yourself get through it, whatever it takes. Even if that means "letting down" the expectations of someone who has other ideas about how you should go about it or spend your time. Once you have survived the journey and have reached a leveling ground, those aspects of your life that, for a time, you have put on the back bench can be reclaimed. You will have time for that; you will not miss anything. Your friends and loved ones, if they are true, will give you either the space or support you need and will not judge you. Those who do wag fingers must be graciously ignored.

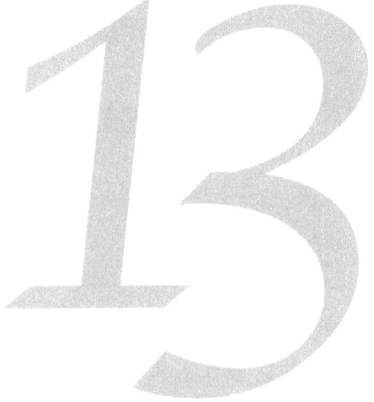

Develop a Hobby

I have found that during the lonely moments when I was trying to "hold steady" having a hobby proved helpful. In my case, I spent many hours working on a miniature art gallery I created from a dollhouse my late-grandfather made for me and gave me on my sixth birthday. In addition to painting and renovating the interior, at the same time I was soliciting art work to display inside. I also created my own miniature art work, and I made a miniature garden for the patio of the miniature gallery as well. All of this activity, by worldly standards, could be deemed trivial and meaningless (what is the point of a dollhouse art gallery?). But this quirky eccentric hobby saved my life during the long lonely hours when my brain was misfiring and my nerves waged war inside my mind. Even as I worked on it, there were times when I myself thought *What is the point of this??* Yet still

I worked, inch by inch, piece by piece, room by room, a little here, a little there. The end has been a thing of beauty, filled with detail, color, creativity, and balance – undertaken all when in my mind I felt everything that is opposite to this: pain, dullness, drabness, lethargy, and disequilibrium.

Any hobby will do. You simply need "something to do" when you are incapable of anything grand. It could be jigsaw puzzles, or adult coloring, or painting, drawing, whittling, or fixing cars. Gardening is an exceptionally helpful hobby because not only does it render the chance to do comfortingly common things such as planting seeds, or pruning bushes, it also gets you outside into the sun or even the rain, and keeps your blood flowing in the elements. Take a class at a local community college or sign up for a workshop on calligraphy. Anything you can do that will get you outside of your head will help you day by day.

14

Become Mindful of Your Thoughts

I have already alluded to the necessity, during your taper, of monitoring how you feel (keeping a log on a calendar or in a notebook). I want to emphasize it here again. Simply the activity of taking stock and then writing down what symptoms you are exhibiting will in its own way impose a measure of distance between you and them. That small wedge can become ground to stand upon—if only a sliver—to enable you to take another inch. That sliver will prove sufficient to help you gain the upper hand when you are feeling over-whelmed. This was the case for me when, nearing the point of breaking down during my second attempt (noted in Chapter 8), I read the entries and objectively assessed my deterioration and thus had the good sense to get help and do something to change course. I could do this because of the unprejudiced analysis of the day-to-day entries of my symptoms and my resultant emotional state. I saw clearly that my symptoms had grown steadily worse and that there were fewer and fewer "windows" or breaks from them. Being able to assess that my situation was worsening instead of improving, enabled me to take necessary steps toward helping myself. It may for a time have the feel of a circuitous route, but the important thing is to keep moving forward, if only by the inch. Self-assessment and self-awareness is the key to your advancement. It is up to you to keep yourself going by checking in with yourself and taking stock.

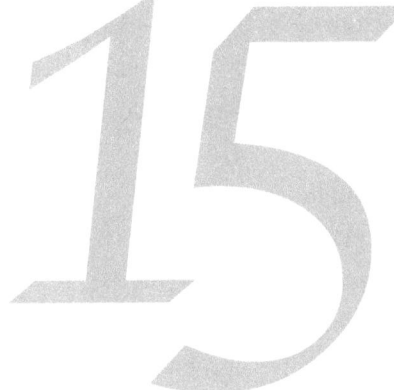

Cultivate
Your Interior Life

You will be called upon to be your own coach and talk yourself through the darkest turns. This touches upon an aspect of this process which, on the one hand, delves into personal and individual sensibilities, but which, on the other hand, I have found to be indispensable for gaining the victory in the struggle to be free of antidepressants. By this I mean the importance of work on the interior life, call it prayer, devotion, meditation – whatever way this important interior work manifests itself in your individual sense of fidelity. It involves intentionality and will, and time to sit still.

There were many, many moments during this struggle when I cried out to God. I remember one occasion in particular when, after two failed attempts to get off the meds and preparing to try yet again, I was walking on a tread mill, feeling exhausted from the effort, aching from the residual chemicals in my system and despairing that I shall ever be free. I felt myself walking, walking, walking while getting nowhere – the experience of the treadmill was also the picture of my life while trying to be rid of antidepressants. I cried out to God: "How long, O Lord? Can you hear me? I am trying. *Please help me.*"

In the moments after speaking those words I will not suggest that the heavens opened and that my face began to shine. The heavens didn't open and the only shine on my face was sweat from the walking as I struggled on, pounding out step after step on that infernal machine. Yet inexplicably there was a measure of consolation that came over me. It was as subtle as it was inexplicable. I had surrendered my course to God, trusted in his help, and kept walking. I read once of a person who asked a spiritual teacher, "What is the road to heaven?" The teacher answered, "Keep walking – that is the shortest road."[2]

So much of the success of the taper will stand or fall on the ability to be patient, to keep trying, to believe and to hope, and ultimately to continue on. All of these invisible aspects—patience, effort, belief, hope—are summoned and realized inside the our minds and souls. The help we receive when we focus upon them and pray or ponder them is like the work of the herbs or the tinctures or nutrition or even the exercise we get as we fortify ourselves for this long journey. The work of these aspects is subtle, slow, often invisible but ever-present and ultimately powerful. It brings to mind the words of the Trappist monk, Thomas Merton, who wrote "the tree bares her blossoms in silence."

There are also practical habits that can be cultivated to lend ballast to the interior work of healing. During the years of my taper, for example, every night before I turned out the light I took out a notebook and wrote down four moments or events of that day for which I was thankful. I called it my "thankful journal." I chose to cite four things, as opposed to the standard three, because rhythms of thinking often default to "threes" (a three-point sermon; top three priorities and so on). It takes a little more effort and sometimes some real focus to come up with that fourth thing. There were times during the writing of these entries when I struggled to come up with something. But even amid those moments, if you think about it, there exists a landscape blessing for which to give thanks.

For example, on a day in October I wrote down the following thoughts:

"Thankful: 1. Warmth of morning coffee; 2. A warm room and soft bed to come home to; 3. The sound of other people's footsteps; 4. The ability to work."

On another day I wrote:

"Thankful: 1. A man waved to me today as I turned right onto the road—he was walking his dog—a complete stranger; 2. Peace & tranquility of working in the greenhouse; 3. Harvested tomatoes, peppers, beets, & basil; 4. Late afternoon in the greenhouse with the sun luminescing off the moistened leaves."

Even amid the darkest hardest most gutting-wrenching battles of discontinuation, within an inch of you there is a universe of blessing. Do you have hands with which to write? Do you have eyes with which to see? Are you lying in a bed? Are you warm? Are you safe? It takes intentionality to see it and this intentionality will again give you ground to stand upon as, inch by inch, you make the advance in the struggle to get off these drugs.

In the Christian tradition the "greatest commandment" as uttered by Jesus to his followers is to "love the Lord your God with all your heart, and with all your soul, and with all your mind." (Matthew 22:37). Of those three, the mind is the territory of the will – it is, to some degree, able to be worked on, exercised, imposed upon. For the patient trying to win the battle of getting off these mind-battering meds, the mind is the battleground. Impulses assail that arise from the damage done but upon which, if we are patient, we can impose a staying aspect. We can mount an opposition simply by the choice to do something else with our minds. To try.

Help is all around. And the way to get to it is to stop listening to the voices of death that echo within and help yourself. Pull yourself up to mount your own rescue. Only you can do it because only you are in the battle. But once you have done that little bit, there is a universe of help, visible and invisible, to carry you the rest of the way. You have to believe it. You have to be ready to die believing it.

2. Francis de Sales, *The Art of Loving God,* Sophia Institute Press (1998), p. 93.

A Final Word

The biggest sorrow I have carried in this struggle is the loss of that part of me that used to ignite a spark of passion about ideas, issues, and more so, God. This spark would awaken my pen and formulate in my mind an entire feature-length article or even a book, which I could lay out in my mind before putting pen to paper. These projects often wrote themselves. In fact, there was a time when I was so filled with passion and ideas that I would be writing a book at the same time when I would be working on a major feature article. I could not find enough to write about.

Whatever inner spark incited that kind of proliferation died somewhere along the line during this struggle. There are times now when I can barely write a substantive email. The part of me that defined me and gave expression to my vocation has been lost somewhere through all this. This has caused me great sorrow and I lament on my bed about it.

Yet I consider sometimes whether this loss is altogether a bad thing. Looking back I perceive there may have been a degree of formulaism to the articles and books I wrote. If there is anything these post-divorce and antidepressant-filled years have clarified for me it is the utter superfluousness of articulating life formulaically. So I sometimes ponder whether or not the loss of the elusive "spark" has been a bad thing – causing all the formulae and Christian prescriptions to fade into acquiescence, if perplexed acquiescence.

So far, for me that spark has not returned. I have reckoned with the fact that if I am to carry on in my vocation as a writer, I must carry on without it. It is all right. It is important to keep pressing forward with positive aspirations.

This was a critical lesson I learned during the period of tapering and in the aftermath of discontinuation. That is the value of occupying oneself with positive counter-pursuits as a means to diminish the edges of the abyss. Such pursuits include helping the body (health, nutrition, vigor), nourishing the mind (reading, crossword puzzles) and cultivating the spirit – prayer, meditation, pursuing virtue. "When we are beset by any particular vice, it is well as far as possible to make the opposite virtue your special aim. . . . Thus, if I am beset with pride or anger, I must above all else strive to cultivate humility and gentleness."[3] In this way, if we survive it, our struggle with discontinuation can become a grace – and not a grace only, but a grace that saves and sanctifies.

3. Francis de Sales, *Introduction to the Devout Life*, Vintage; 1st edition (2002), p 88.

Addenda

Helpful "Things to Do" when Tapering

- Keep a journal
- Plan a garden and research it; then plant it
- Go for a walk
- Take up painting or drawing
- Start an adult coloring book
- Write a thank you note to someone, thanking him or her for even the simplest thing
- Take a class on calligraphy
- Breathe in fresh air
- Listen to running water
- Sit outdoors by a fire-pit, watching the flames and listening to the night sounds
- Take a hot shower or a warm bath

- Get a massage
- Snuggle with a pet
- Burn a scented candle
- Keep a "Thankful Journal"
- Lie down where the afternoon sun streams in a window
- Listen to music
- Spend time in nature
- Go on a lunch date with a good friend
- Call someone
- Pray

About Supplements

Please note: *This information is not intended to be medical advice. Please research all supplements thoroughly before making the decision to begin taking them.*

L-Tryptophan or 5-HTP (5-hydroxytryptophan)

5-HTP is made from the seeds of an African plant called *Griffonia simplicifolia* and is a chemical that the body makes from tryptophan, an essential amino acid that you get from food (such as turkey). After L-tryptophan is converted into 5-HTP, which is then converted to serotonin, the neurotransmitter that relays signals between brain cells described in Chapter 4. 5-HTP helps raise serotonin levels in the brain, which may help regulate mood. 5-HTP may have a positive effect on sleep, mood, anxiety, appetite, and pain sensation.[4]

Other helpful supplements

Other supplements that may help your body navigate that tenuous passage through the lower doses include activated charcoal (to purge toxins from your system), fish oils or krill oil (to increase brain functionality); glutathione (GSH); melatonin; magnesium; vitamin B Complex; L-tyrosine or L-phenylalanine (DLPA;) Himalayan salt or sea salt.

St. John's Wort is a plant-based antidepressant that is known to help normalize serotonin levels during withdrawal. If you don't find the 5-HTP or the L-tryptophan helpful, this could be another option. It has been tested in clinical trials and has proven itself as one of the only herbal treatments for mild cases of depression.

4. In 1989 an outbreak of eosinophilic myalgia syndrome was traceable to what researchers thought then was contaminated L-tryptophan resulting in the U.S. Food and Drug Administration pulling tryptophan supplements off the market. Since then, research has advanced and the link between this anomalous outbreak and L-tryptophan has been questioned. There is no longer any alert related to its use and it is deemed a "safe and effective amino acid." See "L-Tryptophan: It's Back, It's Safe & It's Effective – Informed Opinion," Gene Bruno, MS, MHS, Natural Health Research Institute, http://www.natural-healthresearch.org/l-tryptophan-back-safe-effective.

Prayers for Healing and Recovery

1.

*Our Father, help me to believe this day that there is a
power to lift me up which is
stronger than all the things that hold me down. Amen.*
(George Buttrick)

2.

*If you send me rest, I will rest in You. Let me rest in
Your will and be silent. Amen.*
(Thomas Merton)

3.

*It is you, Lord, that keeps the lamp of my hopes still
burning; shine on the darkness about me. Amen.*
(Saint Augustine)

*Lord, support me all the day long until the shadows
lengthen and the evening comes and the busy world is
hushed and the fever of life is over
and our work is done. Amen.*
(Saint Francis of Assisi)

4.

*Deep peace of the running wave to you,
Deep peace of the flowing air to you,
Deep peace of the quiet earth to you,
Deep peace of the shining stars to you,
Deep peace of the Son of Peace to you, forever.
Amen.*
(Scottish Prayer)

5.

We ask you, Master, be our helper and defender.
Rescue those in distress; raise up the fallen; assist the
needy; heal the sick; turn back those of your people
who stray; feed the hungry; release our captives; revive
the weak; encourage those who lose heart. Amen.
(Clement of Rome, attributed)

6.

O Eternal and most gracious God,
though you suffered some dimness,
some clouds of sadness
to shed themselves upon my soul,
I humbly bless your Holy Name, that you have afford-
ed me the light of your Spirit against which the prince of
darkness cannot prevail nor hinder your illumination in
our darkest night. Amen.
(John Donne)

7.

I have found and have known, by your great mercy,
that the love of a man's heart that has been abandoned
and broken and poor is most pleasing to you and at-
tracts the gaze of your pity, and that it is your desire and
your consolation to be very close to those who love you
and call upon you. Amen.
(Thomas Merton)

8.

Depart, O ye unfruitful wind,
which parcheth up my soul,
and come,
O gracious south wind,
blow upon my garden.
Amen.
(Francis de Sales)

9.

Lord, be with me this day,
Within me to purify me;
Above me to draw me up;
Beneath me to sustain me;
Before me to lead me;
Behind me to restrain me;
Around me to protect me. Amen.
(Saint Patrick)

10.

Go securely and in peace,
my blessed soul.
The One who created and made you holy
has always loved you tenderly as a mother her dear
child.
And you, Lord, are blessed
because You have created me.
Amen.
(Clare of Assisi)

About Wendy Murray

Wendy Murray has enjoyed a distinguished career as a national award-winning journalist and author. She writes this short book as one who has contended in the arena of the struggle of depression, the debilitating effects of antidepressants and the anguish involved in getting off of them. She has launched a website – Surviving SSRIs – to support those suffering from the harsh effects of antidepressants and those suffering in their attempt to quit them. She is the author of several books, including *A Mended and Broken Heart, the Life and Love of Francis of Assisi* (Basic Books) and a novel, *The Warrior King* (Ecco Qua Press).

Personal Notes

Personal Notes

Personal Notes

Personal Notes

Personal Notes

Personal Notes

Personal Notes

Personal Notes

Personal Notes

Personal Notes

www.ingramcontent.com/pod-product-compliance
Lightning Source LLC
Chambersburg PA
CBHW031253280526
45784CB00004B/1842